LIVING WITH SPINAL STENOSIS

A Guide To Managing The Condition

Burley Brown

i

Table of Contents

Introduction

Welcome to "Living with Spinal Stenosis: A Guide to Managing the Condition." This comprehensive book aims to provide you with valuable insights, practical advice, and helpful strategies for navigating the challenges associated with spinal stenosis. Whether you have recently been diagnosed or have been living with this condition for some time, this guide empowers you with knowledge and helps you take control of your life.

Spinal stenosis is a common condition that affects the spinal canal, causing narrowing and putting pressure on the spinal cord and nerves. This can lead to various symptoms, such as back pain, numbness, weakness, and difficulties with mobility. It can significantly impact your daily activities, mobility, and overall quality of life. However, with the proper understanding, management techniques, and support, it is possible to lead a fulfilling life despite the challenges posed by spinal stenosis.

In this book, we will delve into the intricacies of spinal stenosis, exploring its causes, symptoms, and different types. We will discuss various treatment options, both non-surgical and surgical, providing a comprehensive understanding of what choices are available to you and how they can alleviate your symptoms. Additionally, we will explore the importance of self-care, lifestyle modifications, and preventive measures that can help you manage flare-ups and maintain a healthy spine.

We understand that living with spinal stenosis can be physically and emotionally demanding. Therefore, we will also address the psychological aspects of coping with chronic pain, stress, and emotional well-being, offering guidance on seeking support and maintaining a positive mindset throughout your journey.

Moreover, this guide recognizes the importance of adapting your living environment to accommodate your needs. We will provide practical advice on home modifications, assistive devices, and creating a supportive work environment to promote accessibility and ease your daily life.

The book contains informative illustrations, practical tips, and personal anecdotes from individuals who have successfully managed spinal stenosis. We have also included a comprehensive FAQ section to address common questions and concerns that you may have.

Remember, this guide is not a substitute for professional medical advice but a companion to assist you in understanding and managing spinal stenosis. By arming yourself with knowledge, implementing effective strategies, and seeking appropriate medical guidance, you can reclaim control over your life and continue to pursue a fulfilling and active lifestyle.

Let us embark on this journey together, empowering ourselves and fostering a sense of resilience as we navigate the challenges of living with spinal stenosis.

Understanding Spinal Stenosis

Spinal stenosis is characterized by the narrowing the spinal canal, which houses the spinal cord and nerve roots. The spinal canal, a hollow space within the spine, provides protection and allows the passage of nerves that transmit signals between the brain and the body. When the spinal canal narrows, it can pressure the spinal cord and nerves, leading to various symptoms.

Causes and Risk Factors

Spinal stenosis can have multiple causes. One common cause is the natural aging process, known as degenerative changes, where the spinal structures gradually deteriorate. This can include the breakdown of intervertebral discs, the growth of bone spurs (osteophytes), and the thickening of ligaments in the spine.

Other factors that can contribute to spinal stenosis include

Herniated discs: When the discs between the vertebrae bulge or rupture, they can encroach upon the spinal canal.

Bone overgrowth: Certain conditions, such as osteoarthritis, can cause the growth of bone spurs that narrow the spinal canal.

Spinal injuries: Trauma to the spine, such as fractures or dislocations, can lead to spinal stenosis.

Congenital conditions: Some individuals may have a narrower spinal canal, increasing their susceptibility to spinal stenosis.

Genetic factors: Certain genetic traits can predispose individuals to develop spinal stenosis.

Types of Spinal Stenosis

Spinal stenosis can occur in different spine regions, leading to specific symptoms and treatment approaches. The two main types are:

2

Cervical stenosis occurs when the spinal canal in the neck region narrows, affecting the spinal cord. Cervical stenosis can result in symptoms such as neck pain, weakness or numbness in the arms, and difficulties with coordination or balance.

Lumbar stenosis: Lumbar stenosis involves the narrowing of the spinal canal in the lower back, which can put pressure on the nerve roots. Symptoms may include lower back pain, radiating leg pain (sciatica), weakness or numbness in the legs, and cramping or fatigue with walking or standing.

Symptoms and Diagnosis

The symptoms of spinal stenosis can vary depending on the location and severity of the narrowing. Some common signs and symptoms include:

- Pain or discomfort in the affected spine area, such as the back, neck, buttocks, or legs.

- Numbness, tingling, or a "pins-and-needles" sensation in the extremities.
- Weakness or muscle cramping in the arms or legs.
- Difficulties with balance, coordination, or walking, particularly in lumbar stenosis cases.

To diagnose spinal stenosis, your healthcare provider typically begins with a thorough medical history assessment and physical examination. They may evaluate your symptoms, range of motion, muscle strength, and reflexes and conduct various tests to confirm the diagnosis. These tests may include X-rays, magnetic resonance imaging (MRI), computed tomography (CT) scans, or electromyography (EMG) to evaluate nerve function.

By understanding spinal stenosis's definition, causes, types, and symptoms, you can gain insight into this condition's complexities and better communicate with healthcare professionals about your specific experiences. In the following sections, we will explore treatment options, self-care strategies, and other aspects of managing spinal stenosis to empower you with the knowledge and tools needed to navigate this condition effectively.

The Anatomy of the Spine

Structure and Function of the Spine

To understand spinal stenosis, it is essential to have a basic understanding of the structure and function of the spine. The spine, also known as the vertebral column or backbone, is a complex and intricate system that provides support, stability, and protection for the spinal cord.

The spine is composed of bones called vertebrae stacked on top of one another. In the adult human spine, there are typically 33 vertebrae, divided into five regions: cervical (neck), thoracic (upper back), lumbar (lower back), sacral (pelvic area), and coccygeal (tailbone).

Between each pair of vertebrae, intervertebral discs act as shock absorbers and allow for flexibility and movement. These discs comprise a tough outer layer called the annulus fibrosus and a gel-like inner core called the nucleus pulposus.

The spinal canal, located in the center of the vertebrae, houses the spinal cord. The spinal cord is a long, cylindrical bundle of nerves that extends from the base of the brain down to the lower back. It carries sensory information from the body to the brain and transmits motor signals from the brain to the muscles.

Nerve roots branch out from the spinal cord at each vertebral level through small openings called neural foramina. These nerve roots then join to form the peripheral nerves that extend to different body areas, enabling sensation and movement.

How Spinal Stenosis Affects the Spine

In spinal stenosis, the narrowing of the spinal canal or neural foramina can cause compression and pressure on the spinal cord or nerve roots. This can lead to a range of symptoms, depending on the location and severity of the stenosis.

When the spinal canal narrows, it restricts the space available for the spinal cord, potentially leading to compression and irritation. The pressure on the spinal cord can disrupt the normal functioning of the nerves, resulting in symptoms such as pain, numbness, weakness, and difficulties with coordination.

Similarly, if the neural foramina narrow, it can impinge on the nerve roots as they exit the spine. This can cause radiating pain, tingling, or weakness in the areas supplied by those specific nerves. For example, in lumbar stenosis, compression of the nerve roots in the lower back may lead to symptoms that radiate down the legs, commonly known as sciatica.

It's worth noting that spinal stenosis can develop gradually over time as the spinal structures degenerate or due to other contributing factors. The narrowing may progress slowly, and symptoms may worsen gradually as the condition advances.

Understanding the intricate anatomy of the spine and how spinal stenosis affects its structures can provide insight into the underlying mechanisms of this condition. In the subsequent sections, we will explore treatment options, self-care strategies, and lifestyle modifications that can help manage spinal stenosis and alleviate its associated symptoms.

Treatment Options

When managing spinal stenosis, the treatment approach is tailored to the individual's condition, symptoms, and overall health. The primary goal of treatment is to relieve pain, reduce pressure on the spinal cord or nerve roots, and improve functional abilities. Here are some standard treatment options for spinal stenosis:

Non-Surgical Approaches

Medications: Pain management is often achieved through the use of medications. Nonsteroidal anti-inflammatory drugs (NSAIDs), such as ibuprofen or naproxen, can help reduce inflammation and alleviate pain. In some cases, muscle relaxants or medications that target nerve pain (such as gabapentin or pregabalin) may be prescribed.

Physical Therapy: A structured physical therapy program can be beneficial in strengthening the muscles surrounding the spine, improving flexibility, and enhancing posture and body mechanics. Physical therapists may incorporate exercises, stretches, manual therapy techniques, and modalities like heat or cold therapy into the treatment plan.

Epidural Steroid Injections: The healthcare provider may sometimes recommend epidural steroid injections. These injections deliver a combination of corticosteroid medication and a local anesthetic directly into the affected area of the spine. They can help reduce inflammation and provide temporary pain relief.

Assistive Devices: The use of assistive devices can assist in relieving symptoms and improving mobility. For example, a back brace or lumbar corset can provide support and stability to the spine. Canes or walkers may be utilized to help with balance and reduce strain on the spine during walking.

Alternative Therapies: Some individuals find relief from spinal stenosis symptoms through alternative therapies, such as acupuncture, chiropractic care, or massage therapy. These modalities may help alleviate pain, reduce muscle tension, and improve overall well-being.

Surgical Interventions

Decompressive Surgery: Surgical intervention may be considered if non-surgical methods do not provide sufficient relief, or if the condition is severe and significantly impacts daily functioning. Decompressive surgeries aim to alleviate pressure on the spinal cord or nerve roots by removing the structures causing the narrowing. Standard procedures include laminectomy, laminotomy, or foraminotomy.

Spinal Fusion: In some cases, spinal fusion may be necessary to stabilize the spine after decompressive surgery or to address conditions such as spinal instability or deformity. Spinal fusion involves fusing two or more vertebrae using bone grafts, screws, rods, or cages. This restricts movement in the fused segment, reducing pain and providing stability.

Additionally, self-care strategies, lifestyle modifications, and preventive measures can also play a significant role in managing spinal stenosis. These aspects will be discussed in detail in the upcoming sections, providing a comprehensive understanding of living with and managing this condition effectively.

Self-Care and Lifestyle Modifications

While medical interventions are crucial in managing spinal stenosis, incorporating self-care strategies and lifestyle modifications can significantly contribute to symptom relief and overall well-being. Here are some self-care practices and lifestyle adjustments that can help individuals with spinal stenosis:

Physical Activity and Exercise

Regular physical activity is essential for maintaining overall health and managing spinal stenosis. Exercise can help strengthen the muscles supporting the spine, improve flexibility, and promote proper posture. However, choosing low-impact activities that minimize stress on the spine is essential. Recommended exercises for individuals with spinal stenosis may include:

Walking: Walking is a low-impact aerobic exercise that helps improve cardiovascular health and promotes gentle spine movement.

14

Swimming or Water Aerobics: Exercising in water provides buoyancy and reduces joint and spine stress. Swimming or water aerobics can be beneficial for strengthening muscles and improving range of motion.

Cycling: Riding a stationary bike or using a recumbent bike can provide a cardiovascular workout without putting excessive strain on the spine.

Stretching and Gentle Yoga: Gentle stretching exercises and yoga poses can help improve flexibility, relieve muscle tension, and enhance posture.

It is essential to consult with a healthcare professional or physical therapist to determine the most appropriate exercise program tailored to your specific needs and limitations.

Posture and Body Mechanics

- Practicing good posture and body mechanics can help alleviate strain on the spine and reduce symptoms of spinal stenosis. Here are some tips for maintaining proper posture:

- When sitting, use a chair with good lumbar support and sit with your feet flat on the floor. Avoid slouching or crossing your legs for extended periods.
- When standing, distribute your weight evenly on both feet, keep your shoulders back, and avoid excessive leaning or slumping forward.
- When lifting heavy objects, bend your knees and lift with your legs rather than your back. Avoid twisting or jerking motions while lifting.

Weight Management

Maintaining a healthy weight is essential for managing spinal stenosis. Excess weight stresses the spine, exacerbating symptoms and accelerating degenerative changes. By adopting a balanced diet and engaging in regular physical activity, individuals can achieve and maintain a healthy weight, reducing the burden on the spine.

Pain Management Techniques

Various pain management techniques can provide relief from the discomfort associated with spinal stenosis. These may include:

Applying heat or cold packs: Heat therapy, such as a heating pad or warm bath, can help relax muscles and alleviate pain. Cold or ice packs applied to the affected area can reduce inflammation and temporarily numb the area.

Over-the-counter pain medications: Nonsteroidal anti-inflammatory drugs (NSAIDs), such as ibuprofen or naproxen, can help reduce pain and inflammation. However, consulting with a healthcare professional before taking any medication is essential to ensure it is safe and appropriate for you.

Relaxation techniques: Techniques like deep breathing exercises, meditation, or guided imagery can help relax the body and reduce stress, contributing to pain relief.

Assistive Devices and Ergonomic Modifications

Using assistive devices and ergonomic modifications can help individuals with spinal stenosis manage their symptoms more effectively. Examples include:

Lumbar cushions or pillows can provide additional support and promote proper spinal alignment when sitting for extended periods.

Ergonomic chairs and workstations: Using ergonomic chairs and adjusting workstations to maintain proper posture and reduce strain on the spine can benefit individuals with desk jobs.

Orthotic devices: Custom orthotic devices, such as shoe inserts or orthopedic braces, may help provide support and stability to the spine and improve gait.

Stress Management and Emotional Well-being

Living with a chronic condition like spinal stenosis can have emotional and psychological impacts. Managing stress and promoting emotional well-being is essential. Engaging in activities that bring joy, practicing relaxation techniques, seeking support from loved ones or support groups, and considering therapy or counseling can all contribute to better overall mental health.

By implementing these self-care strategies and making lifestyle modifications, individuals with spinal stenosis can improve their quality of life, reduce pain, and enhance their ability to engage in daily activities. However, consulting with healthcare professionals and receiving personalized guidance based on your specific condition and needs is essential.

Preventing and Managing Flare-Ups

Flare-ups of symptoms are common for individuals with spinal stenosis, but some preventive measures and strategies can help manage and minimize these episodes. By being proactive and implementing the following techniques, individuals can reduce the frequency and severity of flare-ups:

Maintaining a Healthy Lifestyle

A healthy lifestyle plays a crucial role in preventing and managing flare-ups. Here are some key aspects to focus on:

Regular Exercise: Engaging in regular low-impact exercises, as recommended by a healthcare professional or physical therapist, helps keep the spine strong, flexible, and well-supported. Stick to a consistent exercise routine that includes stretching, strengthening, and aerobic activities.

Balanced Diet: Eating a well-balanced diet rich in nutrients can support overall health and provide the body with the necessary resources for healing and optimal functioning. Include a variety of fruits, vegetables, lean proteins, whole grains, and healthy fats in your meals.

Adequate Sleep: Prioritize getting enough quality sleep as it allows the body to rest and rejuvenate. Create a sleep-friendly environment, practice good sleep hygiene, and establish a regular sleep schedule.

Stress Management: Stress can exacerbate symptoms and contribute to flare-ups. Find stress-management techniques that work for you, such as deep breathing exercises, meditation, mindfulness, or engaging in hobbies and activities that promote relaxation and enjoyment.

Body Mechanics and Posture

Practicing proper body mechanics and maintaining good posture are essential in preventing strain on the spine. Consider the following guidelines:

Lifting: When lifting objects, use your legs and core muscles, rather than your back, to minimize stress on the spine. Bend at the knees, keep the object close to your body, and avoid twisting or jerking movements.

Sitting: Choose a chair with good lumbar support and sit straight back, shoulders relaxed, and feet flat on the floor. Avoid sitting for prolonged periods and take breaks to stretch and move around.

Standing and Walking: Distribute your weight evenly on both feet while standing. When walking, maintain an upright posture and take regular breaks if needed.

Ergonomics and Workspace Setup

If you have a desk job or spend long hours working on a computer, consider making ergonomic adjustments to your workspace:

Chair and Desk: Ensure your chair provides proper lumbar support, and adjust the height of your desk and chair to maintain a neutral position for your arms and wrists.

Monitor Placement: Position your computer monitor at eye level to avoid straining your neck and upper back. Use a document holder to keep reference materials at a comfortable viewing angle.

Keyboard and Mouse: Keep your keyboard and mouse at a height that allows your wrists to remain neutral, and use a wrist rest if needed.

Pacing and Rest

Learning to pace yourself and avoid overexertion can help prevent flare-ups. Listen to your body's signals and take breaks when needed. Avoid prolonged periods of standing, sitting, or engaging in activities that exacerbate your symptoms. Incorporate regular periods of relaxation throughout your day to allow your body to recover.

Communication and Support

Maintaining open communication with your healthcare provider is essential for managing and preventing flare-ups. Discuss any changes in symptoms, concerns, or questions you may have. Additionally, seek support from friends, family, or groups to share experiences, gain insights, and receive emotional support.

Adapting Your Living Environment

Adapting your living environment to accommodate the challenges posed by spinal stenosis can significantly enhance your comfort, mobility, and overall quality of life. Making thoughtful modifications and incorporating assistive devices can help create a safe and supportive space. Consider the following aspects when adapting your living environment:

Home Accessibility

Creating a home environment that promotes accessibility and ease of movement is essential. Here are some modifications to consider:

Clear Pathways: Ensure clear pathways throughout your home, removing any obstacles or clutter that impede movement. This is especially important in high-traffic areas such as hallways and entrances.

Handrails and Grab Bars: Install handrails and grab bars where additional support is needed, such as staircases, bathrooms, and near beds. These fixtures can help with stability and prevent falls.

Bathroom Modifications: Consider installing a raised toilet seat, grab bars near the toilet and shower, and a non-slip mat or adhesive strip in the shower or bathtub. These modifications can enhance safety and accessibility in the bathroom.

Bedroom Adjustments: Make sure your bed is at an appropriate height for easy entry and exit. Consider using a mattress that provides adequate support and comfort. Additionally, arranging your bedroom items within easy reach can minimize strain and promote independence.

Assistive Devices

Incorporating assistive devices into your living environment can make daily tasks more manageable. Here are some examples:

Mobility Aids: Depending on your needs, consider using assistive devices such as canes, walkers, or wheelchairs to improve stability and mobility.

Reaching Tools: Long-handled reaching tools can help you access items on high shelves or the floor without straining your spine. These tools can be handy for tasks like reaching for objects or retrieving clothing.

Adaptive Equipment: Explore adaptive equipment designed to facilitate various activities. For instance, there are specially designed kitchen utensils with larger handles for easier grip and electric appliances that reduce the need for repetitive manual tasks.

Lighting and Home Safety

Optimizing lighting and ensuring a safe living environment is crucial for individuals with spinal stenosis. Consider the following:

Adequate Lighting: Proper lighting helps enhance visibility and reduces the risk of accidents. Ensure that all areas of your home are well-lit, especially staircases, hallways, and work areas.

Non-Slip Surfaces: Use non-slip mats or rugs with rubber backing to prevent slips and falls. Secure loose carpets or remove them altogether to minimize tripping hazards.

Electrical Safety: Arrange electrical cords and cables in a way that reduces the risk of tripping. Consider using cord organizers or tape to keep them secure and out of the way.

Furniture and Ergonomics

Choosing the right furniture and arranging it ergonomically can promote comfort and spinal alignment. Consider the following tips:

Supportive Seating: Opt for chairs and sofas that provide good lumbar support and promote proper posture. Consider using cushions or pillows to add extra support as needed.

Ergonomic Workstations: If you have a home office or work from home, ensure that your desk and chair are ergonomically designed to promote proper posture and reduce strain on your spine. Adjust the height of your chair and desk to align with your body.

Bed Selection: Choose a mattress and pillows that provide adequate support and alignment for your spine. Experiment with different types of mattresses to find the one that suits your needs.

Adapting your living environment to accommodate spinal stenosis can improve your comfort, safety, and overall well-being. Consult healthcare professionals, occupational therapists, or home accessibility experts for personalized advice and recommendations based on your specific needs and home layout.

Emotional and Psychological Well-being

Living with spinal stenosis can significantly impact your emotional and psychological well-being. Chronic pain, physical limitations, and lifestyle adjustments can sometimes lead to feelings of frustration, sadness, or anxiety. It is crucial to prioritize your mental health and seek support when needed. Here are some strategies to promote emotional well-being while managing spinal stenosis:

Education and Understanding

Educating yourself about spinal stenosis can help you better understand the condition and its management. Learning about the causes, symptoms, treatment options, and lifestyle modifications can empower you to take an active role in your care. Consult reputable sources, speak with healthcare professionals, and consider joining support groups or online communities where you can connect with others facing similar challenges.

Expressing Emotions and Seeking Support

It is essential to acknowledge and express your emotions related to spinal stenosis. Share your feelings with trusted friends, family members, or support groups. Sometimes, simply talking about your experiences can provide relief and support. If needed, consider seeking professional help from therapists, psychologists, or counselors specializing in chronic pain management or rehabilitation. They can provide guidance and strategies to cope with the emotional aspects of living with spinal stenosis.

Stress Management Techniques

Managing stress is crucial for your overall well-being. Chronic pain and physical limitations can be stressful and exacerbate symptoms. Consider incorporating stress management techniques into your daily routine:

Relaxation Techniques: Practice deep breathing exercises, meditation, or progressive muscle relaxation to help relax your body and reduce stress.

Mindfulness: Engage in mindfulness exercises to focus on the present moment and cultivate a sense of calm. This can involve mindful walking, mindful eating, or guided imagery.

Hobbies and Activities: Engage in activities that bring you joy and help you relax. It could be reading, listening to music, painting, gardening, or any other activity that helps you unwind and divert your attention.

Social Support and Connection

Maintaining social connections and seeking support from others is vital for your emotional well-being. Stay connected with friends, family, and support groups who can provide understanding, empathy, and encouragement. Sharing your experiences and listening to others who face similar challenges can create a sense of belonging and reduce feelings of isolation.

Positive Thinking and Self-Care

Cultivating a positive mindset and practicing self-care can contribute to your emotional well-being. Here are some suggestions:

Positive Affirmations: Practice positive self-talk and affirmations. Remind yourself of your strengths, resilience, and achievements. Focus on what you can do rather than dwelling on limitations.

Self-Care Activities: Prioritize self-care activities that bring you joy and relaxation. This could include engaging in hobbies, spending time in nature, taking warm baths, practicing self-compassion, or pampering yourself.

Seeking Balance: Find a balance between managing your condition and engaging in activities that promote your overall well-being. Pace yourself, set realistic goals, and listen to your body's signals to prevent overexertion.

Maintaining a Healthy Spine

While spinal stenosis presents challenges, there are steps you can take to maintain a healthy spine and potentially slow down the progression of the condition. By adopting healthy habits and incorporating specific practices into your daily routine, you can support the overall well-being of your spine. Here are some strategies for maintaining a healthy spine:

Exercise and Physical Activity

Regular exercise is essential for maintaining a healthy spine. It can strengthen the supporting muscles, improve flexibility, and promote proper posture. However, choosing safe and appropriate exercises for your condition is essential. Consult your healthcare provider or a physical therapist to develop an exercise plan tailored to your needs. Consider the following types of exercises:

Low-Impact Aerobic Exercises: Walking, swimming, or using an elliptical machine can promote cardiovascular health without placing excessive strain on your spine.

Core-Strengthening Exercises: Engaging in exercises that target the muscles of your abdomen and lower back can help stabilize your spine. Examples include planks, bridges, and gentle Pilates or yoga exercises.

Flexibility Exercises: Stretching exercises can improve flexibility and range of motion in your spine and surrounding muscles. Incorporate gentle stretching routines focusing on your neck, shoulders, back, and legs.

Maintaining Good Posture

Practicing good posture throughout the day can reduce strain on your spine and help prevent further complications. Be mindful of your posture when sitting, standing, and performing daily activities. Here are some tips:

- Sit with your back straight, and shoulders relaxed, and feet flat on the floor. Use a chair that provides adequate support for your lower back.

- When standing, distribute your weight evenly on both feet, keep your shoulders back, and avoid slouching or excessive leaning.
- Use ergonomic equipment, such as an adjustable chair or standing desk, to support proper posture during work or other prolonged activities.
- Be mindful of your posture when lifting objects, bending, or performing household tasks. Bend your knees, keep your back straight, and use your leg muscles to lift rather than strain your back.

Weight Management

Maintaining a healthy weight is crucial for supporting your spine. Excess weight can stress your spine more and exacerbate spinal stenosis symptoms. Strive for a balanced diet and regular physical activity to manage weight effectively. Consult a healthcare professional or nutritionist for personalized guidance on achieving and maintaining a healthy weight.

Quit Smoking

If you smoke, quitting is essential for the overall health of your spine. Smoking reduces blood flow to the spinal discs, contributing to degeneration and back pain. Quitting smoking can improve your spinal health and reduce the risk of further complications.

Regular Medical Check-ups

Regular medical check-ups are essential for monitoring the progress of spinal stenosis and addressing any concerns or changes in symptoms. Work closely with your healthcare provider to develop a comprehensive management plan and ensure your treatment approach is tailored to your needs.

Ergonomics in Daily Activities

Be mindful of your body mechanics and ergonomics when performing daily activities. Whether you are sitting at a desk, lifting heavy objects, or engaging in recreational activities, consider the following:

- Use proper lifting techniques to minimize strain on your spine. Bend your knees, keep the object close to your body, and engage your leg muscles.
- Avoid repetitive motions or activities that place excessive stress on your spine. Take breaks, switch positions, or use assistive devices when needed.
- Make ergonomic adjustments to your workspace, such as adjusting the height of your chair and desk, using proper keyboard and mouse placement, and positioning your computer monitor at eye level.

Living a Fulfilling Life with Spinal Stenosis

Spinal stenosis may present challenges, but it doesn't have to limit your ability to lead a fulfilling and meaningful life. By adopting a positive mindset, making necessary adjustments, and embracing a holistic approach to well-being, you can continue to pursue your passions and find joy in everyday experiences. Here are some strategies for living a fulfilling life with spinal stenosis:

Redefine Your Priorities

Living with spinal stenosis may require you to reassess and adjust your priorities. Take the time to reflect on what truly matters to you and align your activities and goals accordingly. Focus on activities that bring you joy, fulfillment, and a sense of purpose. Whether spending quality time with loved ones, pursuing a hobby, or engaging in creative endeavors, choose activities that enhance your well-being and align with your values.

Stay Engaged and Active

Maintaining an active and engaged lifestyle is essential for physical and mental well-being. Find activities that you can participate in comfortably and modify them as needed. This might involve joining support groups or community organizations, taking up low-impact exercises or sports, or engaging in hobbies that accommodate your physical abilities. Staying connected with others and pursuing your interests can help you maintain a sense of purpose and fulfillment.

Adapt and Modify

Adapting and modifying activities and tasks to suit your physical capabilities can help you overcome challenges and continue enjoying the things you love. Explore adaptive equipment or techniques that can assist you in pursuing your hobbies or daily activities. For example, assistive devices, such as long-handled tools or ergonomic utensils, can make tasks more manageable. Embrace creativity and find innovative ways to adapt your lifestyle to accommodate your condition.

Seek Support

Building a solid support network is crucial for navigating the challenges of spinal stenosis. Seek support from friends, family, and healthcare professionals who can offer encouragement, understanding, and practical assistance. Consider joining support groups or online communities to connect with others with similar experiences. Sharing your journey with others and learning from their experiences can provide a sense of belonging and inspire you to overcome obstacles.

Practice Mindfulness and Gratitude

Cultivating mindfulness and gratitude can help you find peace and contentment amidst the challenges of spinal stenosis. Practice being present in the moment, accepting your limitations, and embracing self-compassion. Engage in gratitude exercises, such as keeping a gratitude journal or expressing appreciation for the small joys in life. Focusing on the positive aspects and practicing mindfulness can shift your perspective and help you find fulfillment in the present moment.

Embrace Self-Care

Self-care plays a vital role in maintaining your overall well-being. Prioritize self-care activities that promote relaxation, stress reduction, and physical comfort. This might involve practicing relaxation techniques, engaging in gentle exercises, pampering yourself with a warm bath or massage, or engaging in activities that bring you joy and rejuvenation. Listen to your body, pace yourself, and honor your limitations.

Foster Emotional Resilience

Developing emotional resilience can empower you to navigate the emotional ups and downs accompanying spinal stenosis. Focus on building coping mechanisms, practicing self-compassion, and seeking professional help if needed. Emotional resilience can help you bounce back from setbacks, maintain a positive outlook, and cultivate a fulfilling and meaningful life.

Conclusion

Living with spinal stenosis presents unique challenges, but with the proper knowledge, strategies, and support, you can effectively manage the condition and lead a fulfilling life. This guide has provided valuable information on understanding spinal stenosis, its causes, symptoms, and various treatment options available.

Adopting a holistic approach that encompasses medical treatments, self-care, lifestyle modifications, and emotional well-being can improve your quality of life and maintain a positive outlook.

Throughout this book, we have explored topics such as understanding spinal stenosis, treatment options, self-care and lifestyle modifications, preventing and managing flare-ups, adapting your living environment, emotional and psychological well-being, maintaining a healthy spine, and living a fulfilling life with spinal stenosis. Each section has offered practical advice, tips, and insights to help you navigate the challenges associated with spinal stenosis.

Remember, spinal stenosis is a chronic condition that requires ongoing management. Working closely with your healthcare provider to develop a personalized treatment plan tailored to your needs is essential. Regular medical check-ups, open communication, and proactive self-care efforts are essential to effectively managing the condition.

While spinal stenosis may pose limitations, it doesn't have to define your life. Embrace a positive mindset, seek support from loved ones and support groups, and adapt your lifestyle to accommodate your condition.

Focus on what brings you joy, engage in activities that nourish your physical and emotional well-being, and make necessary adjustments to create a fulfilling life.

Always remember that you are not alone in this journey. Reach out to healthcare professionals, connect with others with similar experiences, and never hesitate to ask questions or seek guidance when needed. With the proper knowledge, support, and determination, you can navigate the challenges of spinal stenosis and live a meaningful and satisfying life.

Wishing you strength, resilience, and a life filled with joy and fulfillment as you embark on this journey of living with spinal stenosis.

Printed in Great Britain
by Amazon